Slim fast diet recipes for women over 50

Slim Fast Diet Made Easy: Wholesome Recipes to Help Women 50+ Achieve Optimal Health

By

VIOLA PECK

Title: [Slim Fast Diet Recipes for Women Over 50]

Table of Contents

Introduction

Chapter One

Importance of slim diet recipes for women over 50

Why a Slim Diet is Important for Women Over 50

Benefits of a Slim Diet for Women Over 50

Chapter Two

 Breakfast Recipes

Blueberry smoothie

Chocolate peanut butter oatmeal

Greek yogurt parfait

Egg white omelette

Banana nut oatmeal

Chapter Three

Lunch Recipes

Grilled chicken salad

Tuna salad

Grilled chicken sandwich

Chapter Four

Dinner Recipes

Grilled salmon with roasted vegetables

Chicken fajitas bowl

Zucchini noodles spaghetti Bolognese

Turkey chili

Grilled chicken with greek salad

Chapter Five

Conclusion

Additional tips for maintaining a slim diet

Benefits of staying consistent with a slim diet

Introduction

Women's metabolisms tend to slow down as they get older, making it more difficult for them to maintain a healthy weight. Women over 50 who may be struggling with hormonal changes, a loss in muscle mass, and other age-related problems may find this particularly difficult. Through a balanced diet and consistent exercise, one can overcome these difficulties and keep a healthy weight.

The Slim Fast diet is a well-liked weight management plan that provides a practical method of regulating portions and caloric consumption. In this diet, two meals a day are swapped out for Slim Fast meal replacement shakes or bars, and the third meal of the day is a nutritious, balanced meal. A variety of snacks and meal replacements are also available from Slim Fast that can be used in conjunction with the regimen.

The Slim Fast diet can be a successful strategy for women over 50 to control their weight and enhance their general health. Women can make sure that they are obtaining the vitamins and minerals they need to preserve their health as they age by taking nutrient-rich meal replacement products and adhering to a balanced meal plan.

We'll look at some of the top Slim Fast diet recipes for ladies over 50 in this article. These recipes are made to offer a choice of wholesome and mouthwatering meal options that can support women in sticking to their weight loss objectives and ensuring that their nutritional needs are met.

CHAPTER ONE

Importance of slim diet recipes for women over 50

Why a Slim Diet is Important for Women Over 50

Women's bodies change significantly as they age, which may have an impact on their health and wellbeing. The slowdown of the metabolism, which can make it harder to maintain a healthy weight, is one of the most significant alterations. This is why keeping a balanced diet that is low in calories and fat is crucial for women over 50. For the following causes, lean diet recipes are crucial for women over 50:

1) **Increased risk of health problems:** An rise in the likelihood that women will experience health issues such high blood pressure, high cholesterol, diabetes, and heart disease as they get older. A

slim diet and maintaining a healthy weight can help lower the chance of developing these diseases.

2) **Slower metabolism:** Women's metabolisms slow down as they become older, causing them to burn less calories than they did when they were younger. As a result, gaining weight is simpler and losing it more difficult. This effect can be mitigated with a calorie-reduced thin diet.

3) **Bone health:** Women over 50 are more likely to develop osteoporosis, a disease that makes bones brittle and feeble. A lean diet full of calcium and vitamin D can support the maintenance of strong bones.

4) **Hormonal changes:** Age-related hormonal imbalance changes in women can result in weight increase, particularly in the midriff. Blood sugar levels can be stabilized and this kind of weight

gain prevented with a slender diet low in refined carbohydrates and sugar.

In general, women over 50 should eat a diet low in fat and high in nutrient-dense foods like fruits, vegetables, lean proteins, and whole grains to preserve their health and lower their chance of acquiring chronic health issues.

Benefits of a Slim Diet for Women Over 50

For women over 50, a slim diet—which is defined as a balanced, nutritious eating plan created to assist in achieving and maintaining a healthy weight—can offer a number of advantages. Here are a few of the main advantages:

- **Reduces the risk of chronic diseases:** Eating a healthy, balanced diet can help lower the chance of developing chronic conditions including diabetes, heart disease, and some types of cancer.

- **Boosts energy levels:** A balanced diet can help increase energy levels and decrease weariness, which is crucial for women over 50 because they may face energy decreases due to aging.

- **Improves bone health:** Women over 50 are more susceptible to the disorder osteoporosis, which weakens bones and raises the risk of fractures. A lean diet with sufficient calcium and vitamin D can assist to strengthen bones and lower the risk of osteoporosis.

- **Enhances mental clarity:** A nutritious diet can also assist improve mental clarity and cognitive function, which is especially advantageous for women over 50, who may experience age-related reductions in cognitive function.

- **Promotes better sleep:** A lean, nutrient-dense diet can assist improve sleep, which is crucial for general health and well-being.

- **Supports healthy weight management:** A balanced and healthy diet can help women over 50 maintain a healthy weight, which can help minimize the risk of a variety of health concerns.

In general, women over 50 can benefit greatly from a slim diet. It can support greater overall wellbeing, physical and mental health, and lower the risk of chronic diseases.

CHAPTER TWO

Breakfast Recipes

The Slim Fast diet is a well-known weight loss plan that includes a balanced dinner as well as meal replacement shakes, bars, and snacks. The diet aims to aid weight loss in women over 50 by limiting calorie intake and encouraging a healthy lifestyle. Breakfast is a critical meal of the day, so it's important to pick one that will give you energy and keep you satisfied until lunch.

Here are some Slim Fast diet breakfast recipes for women over 50:

❖ **Blueberry Smoothie:**

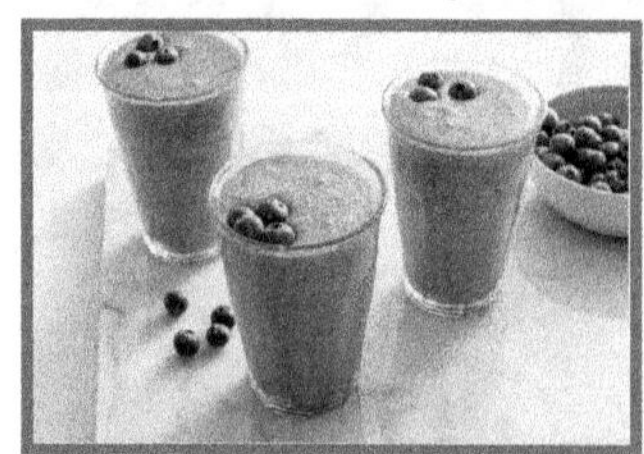

Ingredients:

1 cup of unsweetened almond milk

1 scoop of Slim Fast Vanilla Shake Mix

1 cup of frozen blueberries

1 tbsp of chia seeds

1 tbsp of honey

Instructions:

Combine all ingredients in a blender and blend until smooth.

Pour into a glass and enjoy.

❖ **Chocolate Peanut Butter Oatmeal:**

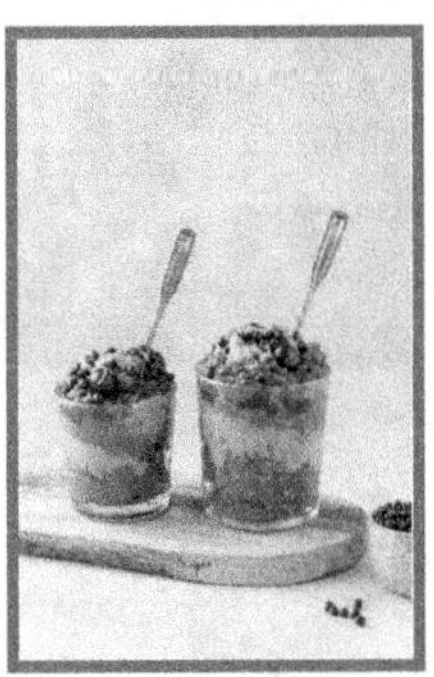

Ingredients:

1 packet of instant oatmeal

1 scoop of Slim Fast Chocolate Shake Mix

1 tbsp of peanut butter

1/2 cup of unsweetened almond milk

1 tsp of honey

Instructions:

Cook oatmeal according to package instructions.

Stir in the Slim Fast Chocolate Shake Mix, peanut butter, and almond milk until well combined.

Drizzle with honey and serve.

❖ **Greek Yogurt Parfait:**

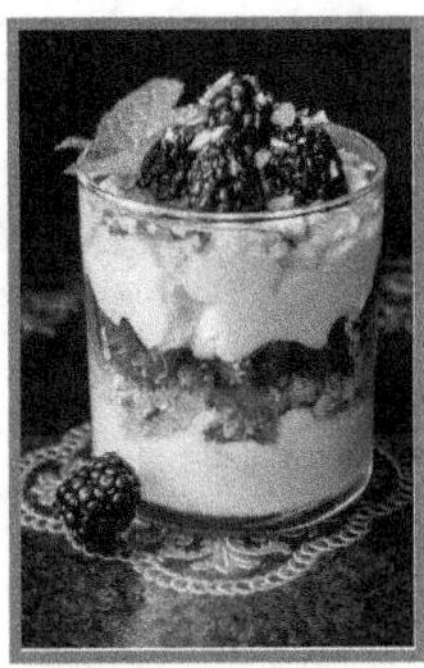

Ingredients:

1 cup of plain Greek yogurt

1 scoop of Slim Fast Vanilla Shake Mix

1/2 cup of mixed berries (strawberries, blueberries, raspberries)

1 tbsp of sliced almonds

1 tsp of honey

Instructions:

In a bowl, mix the Slim Fast Vanilla Shake Mix with the Greek yogurt until well combined.

Layer the yogurt mixture with mixed berries in a glass.

Sprinkle sliced almonds on top and drizzle with honey.

❖ **Egg White Omelet:**

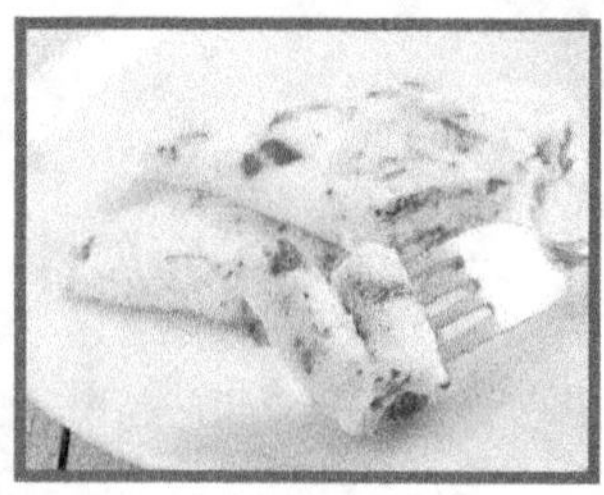

Ingredients:

2 egg whites

1/2 cup of chopped spinach

1/4 cup of diced tomatoes

1/4 cup of diced mushrooms

1/4 cup of diced onions

1/2 oz of low-fat shredded cheddar cheese

1 slice of whole-grain toast

Instructions:

In a non-stick skillet, sauté the spinach, tomatoes, mushrooms, and onions until tender.

In a bowl, whisk the egg whites until frothy.

Pour the egg whites into the skillet and cook until set.

Sprinkle shredded cheese on top and fold the omelet in half.

Serve with a slice of whole-grain toast.

❖ **Banana Nut Oatmeal:**

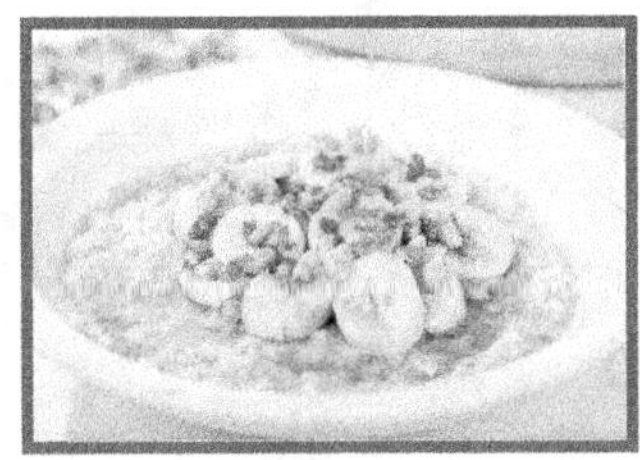

Ingredients:

1 packet of instant oatmeal

1/2 banana, mashed

1 tbsp of chopped walnuts

1 scoop of Slim Fast Vanilla Shake Mix

1/2 cup of unsweetened almond milk

Instructions:

Cook oatmeal according to package instructions.

Stir in the mashed banana, chopped walnuts, Slim Fast Vanilla Shake Mix, and almond milk until well combined.

Serve warm.

These healthy Slim Fast diet breakfast recipes for women over 50 will help them lose weight while giving them the necessary nutrition and energy to tackle the day. They are also simple to prepare. For best outcomes, keep in mind to consume enough of water and include exercise in your regular routine.

CHAPTER THREE

Lunch Recipes

The SlimFast diet is a well-known weight loss plan that entails eating one balanced meal per day, replacing two meals with a meal replacement shake or bar, and nibbling on fruits, vegetables, or SlimFast snacks throughout the day. Through calorie restriction and nutritional and vitamin supplementation, the program seeks to assist people in losing weight.

Maintaining a nutritious diet that is healthful, balanced, and satisfies your needs is crucial for women over 50. Listed below are some lunch meals that fit the SlimFast diet:

- **Grilled Chicken Salad**

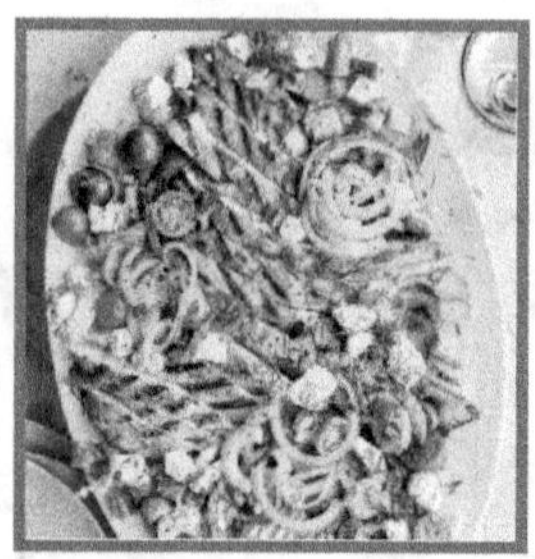

Ingredients:

3 oz grilled chicken breast

2 cups mixed greens

1/2 cup cherry tomatoes

1/2 avocado

1/4 cup sliced red onion

2 tbsp balsamic vinaigrette

Instructions:

Grill chicken breast until cooked through. Mix mixed greens, cherry tomatoes, sliced red onion, and avocado in a bowl. Add grilled chicken to the bowl. Drizzle balsamic vinaigrette over the salad and enjoy!

- **Tuna Salad**

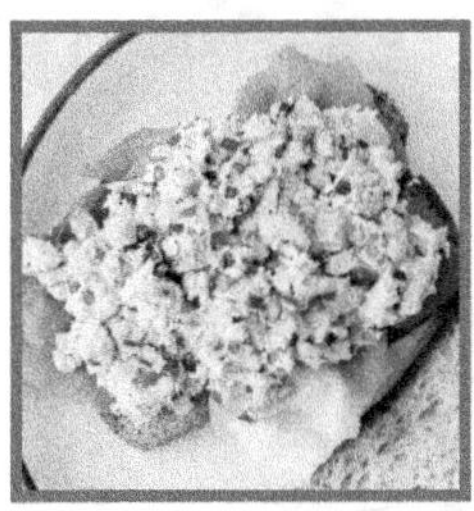

Ingredients:

3 oz canned tuna, drained

1/4 cup chopped celery

1/4 cup chopped red onion

1 tbsp chopped fresh parsley

1 tbsp lemon juice

1 tbsp olive oil

Salt and pepper to taste

Instructions:

Mix canned tuna, chopped celery, chopped red onion, and chopped fresh parsley in a bowl. Drizzle lemon juice and olive oil over the mixture and toss to combine. Season with salt and pepper to taste. Serve the tuna salad on a bed of lettuce or with a side of whole-grain crackers.

- **Grilled Chicken Sandwich**

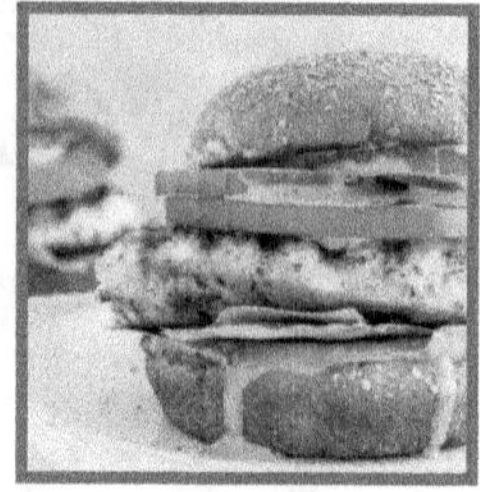

Ingredients:

3 oz grilled chicken breast

1 whole-grain sandwich thin

1 tbsp mayonnaise

1 slice of tomato

1/4 cup shredded lettuce

Salt and pepper to taste

Instructions:

Grill chicken breast until cooked through. Toast the sandwich thin. Spread mayonnaise on one side of the sandwich thin. Add grilled chicken, tomato slice, and shredded lettuce on top of the mayonnaise. Season with salt and pepper to taste. Top with the other half of the sandwich thin and enjoy!

These dishes are created to be high in protein, fiber, and other necessary elements while being low in calories. They are a simple way for women over 50 to have a complete meal while adhering to the SlimFast regimen. Before beginning any weight loss program, it's crucial to speak with a healthcare professional, especially if you have any underlying medical issues.

CHAPTER FOUR

Dinner Recipes

The SlimFast diet is a well-known weight loss plan that instructs dieters to eat SlimFast drinks or meal replacement bars for the first two meals and a nutritious, balanced meal for the third. Many women over 50 who wish to lose weight find this program to be an appealing alternative because it has been developed to be handy and simple to follow.

There are many supper dishes for over-50s on the SlimFast diet that will help you maintain your weight loss objectives while still enjoying a delectable and gratifying meal. Here are some illustrations:

➤ Grilled Salmon with Roasted Vegetables:

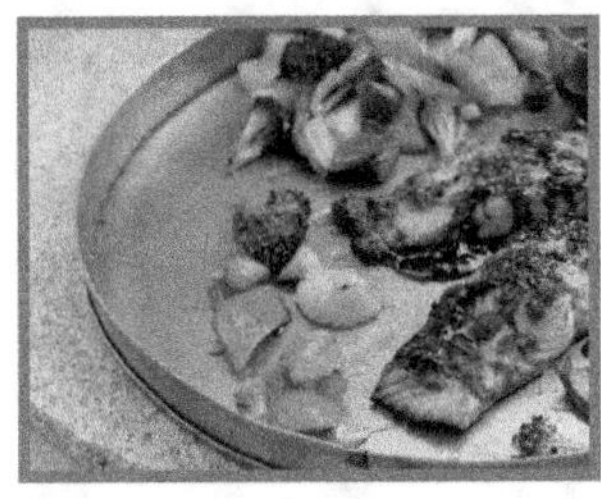

Ingredients:

4 salmon fillets (skin on)

4 cups of mixed vegetables (such as bell peppers, zucchini, onions, and cherry tomatoes)

1 tbsp olive oil

1/2 tsp salt

1/4 tsp black pepper

1/4 tsp garlic powder

1/4 tsp dried oregano

Instructions:

Preheat the oven to 400°F (200°C). Line a baking sheet with parchment paper.

Cut the vegetables into bite-sized pieces and place them on the prepared baking sheet.

Drizzle with olive oil and sprinkle with salt, black pepper, garlic powder, and dried oregano. Toss to coat the vegetables evenly.

Roast the vegetables in the preheated oven for 20-25 minutes, or until they are tender and lightly browned.

While the vegetables are roasting, preheat a grill or grill pan over medium-high heat. Season the salmon fillets with salt and black pepper.

Grill the salmon fllets for 3-4 minutes per side, or until they are cooked through and the skin is crispy.

Serve   the grilled salmon fillets with the roasted vegetables on the side.

> **Chicken Fajita Bowl**

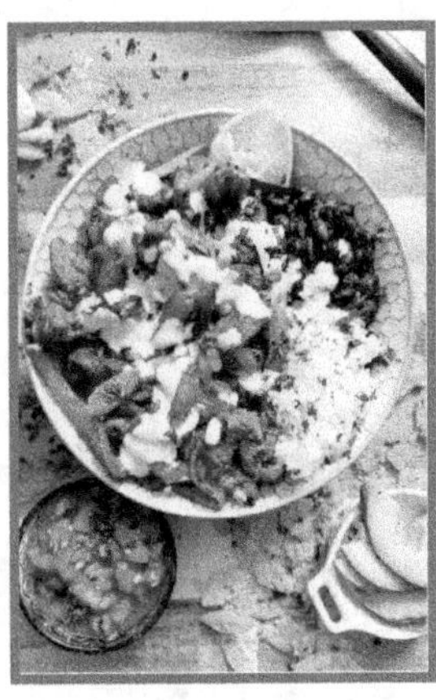

Ingredients:

3 1 tsp each salt, oregano, ground cumin, and garlic powder

2 tsp chili powder

1 tbsp smoked paprika

1 tbsp cornstarch – this isn't a necessary ingredient- it does help spices adhere better to the meat and gives the finished meat a delicious texture

1-1/2 lbs chicken breast or chicken tenders sliced into strips

3 peppers (mix of bell peppers and/or poblano peppers) sliced into thin strips

1 large onion (yellow onion or red onion works just fine) sliced into thin strips

Instructions:

In a skillet over medium-high heat add 1 tsp of olive oil. Once the pan is hot (check by throwing a little water on in if the water sizzles its hot enough) throw the peppers and onions into it, season with salt and pepper, and let them cook until golden brown and soft. When they are done remove from the pan and set aside.

Add two teaspoons of oil into the same skillet over medium-high heat and add the sliced and seasoned fajita chicken. Let it sit (don't move it around or touch it) for about 4-5 minutes. Let it get a nice and golden brown with a nice sear. Then, flip the pieces and let it cook the reset of the way for another few minutes.

Add the peppers back into the chicken and toss together to warm it all up.

> **Zucchini Noodle Spaghetti Bolognese:**

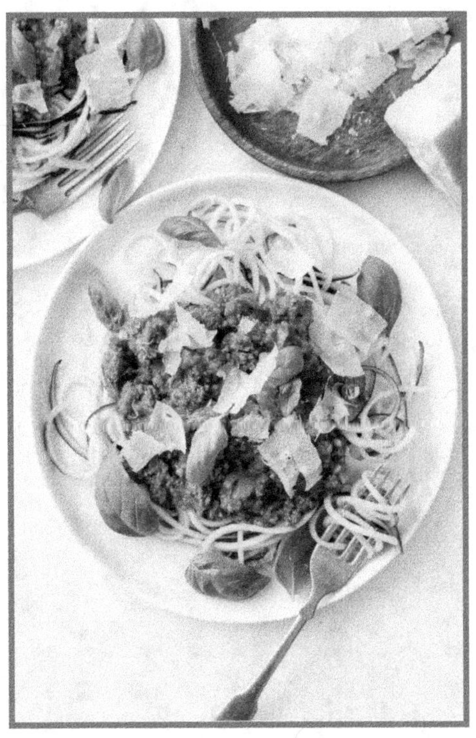

Ingredients:

2 pounds spiralized zucchini (about 4 medium zucchini)

1¾ cups canned crushed tomatoes

2 tablespoons tomato paste

1½ teaspoons white wine vinegar

1/2 teaspoon Italian seasoning

3/4 teaspoon garlic powder

3/4 teaspoon onion powder

1½ teaspoons olive oil

1/4 cup chopped celery

1/4 cup chopped onion

1/4 cup chopped carrots

8 ounces raw extra-lean ground beef (4% fat or less)

1/2 teaspoon salt

1/8 teaspoon black pepper

Instructions:

Bring an extra-large skillet sprayed with nonstick spray to medium-high heat. Cook and stir zucchini until hot and slightly softened, about 3 minutes.

Transfer zucchini to a strainer, and thoroughly drain excess liquid.

In a medium-large bowl, combine crushed tomatoes, tomato paste, vinegar, and Italian seasoning. Add 1/2 teaspoon each garlic powder and onion powder, and mix well.

Drizzle oil in the skillet, and return to medium-high heat. Add celery, onion, and carrots. Cook and stir until slightly softened, about 2 minutes.

Reduce heat to medium. Add beef, and season with salt, pepper, and remaining 1/4 teaspoon each garlic powder and onion powder. Cook, stir, and crumble until veggies have softened and beef is fully cooked, about 5 minutes.

Add tomato mixture to the skillet. Cook and stir until hot and well mixed, about 1 minute.

Add drained zucchini, and cook and stir until hot and well mixed, about 2 minutes.

➤ **Turkey Chili:**

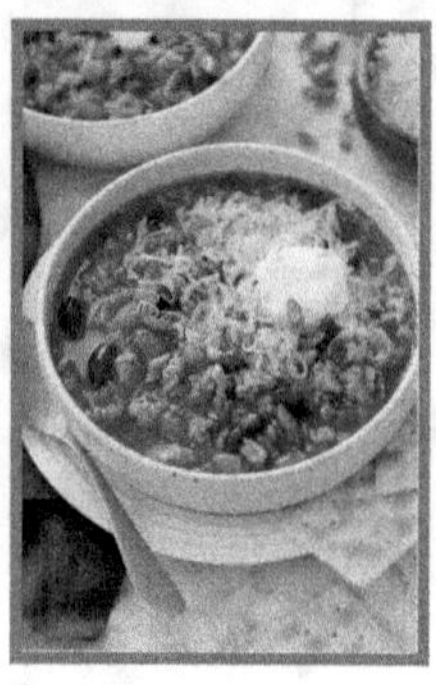

Ingredients:

1 tablespoon olive oil

2 pounds ground turkey, white and dark meat combined

2 cups coarsely chopped onions

2 tablespoons chopped garlic

1 large sweet red pepper, cored, deveined and coarsely chopped

1 jalapeño, cored, deveined and finely chopped

1 tablespoon fresh oregano, chopped, or 1 tablespoon dried 2bay leaves

3 tablespoons chili powder

3 cups canned diced tomatoes

2 cups chicken broth, fresh or canned Salt and black pepper

Instructions:

Heat the oil over high in a large heavy pot and add the turkey meat. Cook until lightly browned, about 5 minutes, chopping down and stirring with the side of a heavy kitchen spoon to break up any lumps.

Add the onions, garlic, sweet pepper, celery, jalapeño, oregano, bay leaves, chili powder and cumin. Stir to blend well. Cook for 5 minutes.

Add the tomatoes, chicken broth, salt and pepper to taste. Bring to a boil, reduce heat and simmer, stirring occasionally, for 15 minutes.

Add the drained beans and cook, stirring occasionally, for 10 minutes longer. Serve in bowls with Cheddar, and sour cream and lime wedges, if desired.

➢ **Grilled Chicken with Greek Salad:**

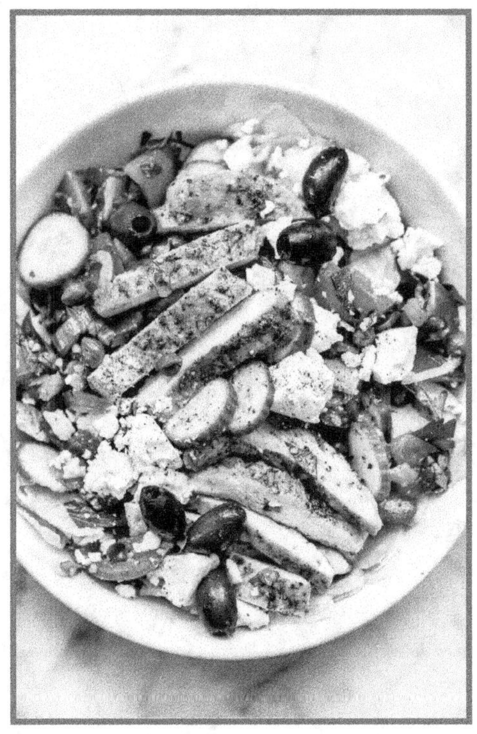

Ingredients:

Romaine lettuce

Chicken breast

Cherry tomatoes

Cucumber

Red onion

Kalamata olives

Feta cheese

Fresh oregano leaves picked (optional)

For the Greek Dressing/marinade

Olive oil

Red wine vinegar

Garlic clove

Dried oregano

Kosher salt

Freshly ground black pepper

Instructions:

Prepare the chicken: First, place the chicken breast in a ziplock bag. Add all the dressing/marinade ingredients to a small jar. Place the lid on and shake well until emulsified. Pour 1/3 of this mixture over the chicken and mix to combine. Keep refrigerated to marinate for at least 1 hour. (if in a rush you can skip marinating the chicken and go right to cooking) Keep remaining 2/3 of the mixture in the jar, refrigerated, to use as a dressing.

Cook Chicken: Then, heat a large non-stick pan or grill pan over medium heat. Add chicken and cook for 8-10 minutes per side, or until the internal temperature reaches 165°F. Transfer the chicken on a place and allow it to sit covered for about 10-12 minutes, then slice it.

Fix the salad bowl: Add the lettuce to a large serving bowl. Top with tomatoes, cucumbers, onion, olives, and sliced chicken. Sprinkle with crumbled feta cheese.
Add dressing: Finally, drizzle the dressing over the salad and toss to combine. Serve immediately and enjoy!

Whatever dinner recipe you come up with, always be mindful of serving sizes and aim for a balanced meal that includes plenty of veggies, lean protein, and healthy fats. Even if you follow the SlimFast regimen, you may still enjoy delicious and satisfying meals and lose weight.

CHAPTER FIVE

Conclusion

In conclusion, the Slim Fast diet can be an option for women over 50 who are looking to lose weight or maintain a healthy weight. However, it is important to approach any diet plan with caution and consult with a healthcare professional before making any significant changes to your diet or lifestyle. While there are many Slim Fast recipes available that can be tailored to individual preferences and dietary needs, it is important to remember that diet alone is not enough for optimal health. Incorporating regular exercise, stress management techniques, and getting enough sleep are also important for overall health and well-being.

Additional Tips for Maintaining a Slim Diet

Maintaining a healthy diet is essential for weight management and overall health. Here are some additional tips for maintaining a slim diet:

Plan your meals: Plan your meals in advance to ensure that you have healthy options available when you're hungry. You can use a meal planner or a food diary to track your food intake and make sure you're eating a balanced diet.

Drink plenty of water: Drinking water can help you feel full and reduce your overall calorie intake. Aim for at least 8-10 glasses of water a day, and consider drinking a glass of water before meals to help you feel full faster.

Eat slowly: Eating slowly can help you feel full faster and reduce your overall calorie intake. Take your time and savor each bite, and try to put your utensils down between bites.

Choose healthy snacks: Choose healthy snacks like fruits, vegetables, nuts, and seeds instead of high-calorie, high-sugar snacks like candy and chips.

Limit processed foods: Processed foods are often high in calories, sugar, and unhealthy fats. Try to limit your intake of processed foods and focus on whole, nutrient-dense foods instead.

Pay attention to portion sizes: Pay attention to portion sizes and try to stick to recommended serving sizes to avoid overeating.

Get enough protein: Protein can help you feel full and reduce your overall calorie intake. Aim for at least 20-30 grams of protein with each meal.

Remember, a healthy diet is not just about what you eat, but also how much you eat and how often you eat. Be mindful of your food choices, listen to your body, and make healthy choices that will help you maintain a healthy weight and feel your best.

Benefits of Staying Consistent with a Slim Diet

Staying consistent with a slim diet can have numerous benefits for your overall health and well-being. Some of the key benefits include:

Weight loss: Consistently following a slim diet can help you lose excess body fat and maintain a healthy weight. This can reduce your risk of many health problems, including heart disease, diabetes, and certain types of cancer.

Improved digestion: Slim diets are often rich in fiber and nutrient-dense foods, which can help improve digestion and promote regularity.

Increased energy: Eating a healthy, balanced diet can provide your body with the nutrients it needs to function optimally, leading to increased energy levels and improved productivity throughout the day.

Better mood: Slim diets that are high in fruits, vegetables, and whole grains have been linked to improved mood and reduced symptoms of depression.

Reduced inflammation: A slim diet that is rich in anti-inflammatory foods can help reduce inflammation in the body, which has been linked to a variety of health problems, including arthritis, heart disease, and cancer.

Overall, staying consistent with a slim diet can help you feel better, look better, and live a healthier, happier life.

Final Thoughts and Encouragement.

If you do decide to try the Slim Fast diet, there are a variety of recipes available that can help keep your meals interesting and satisfying. Additionally, it's important to remember that a sustainable, healthy diet includes a balance of nutrients and should not rely on meal replacement products alone.

For women over 50, it's important to prioritize nutrient-dense foods that support overall health and well-being. This may include incorporating plenty of fruits, vegetables, lean proteins, and healthy fats intoyour diet. Additionally, staying active and getting enough rest can also support a healthy weight and overall health.

Remember to approach any weight loss plan with patience and self-compassion. Making lasting changes to your diet and lifestyle takes time and effort, but with persistence and support, you can achieve your goals.